Copyright 2023

Table of Contents

A disorder in which nerve cell activity in the brain is disturbed, causing seizures.

Epilepsy may occur as a result of a genetic disorder or an acquired brain injury, such as a trauma or stroke.

During a seizure, a person experiences abnormal behavior, symptoms and sensations, sometimes including loss of consciousness. There are few symptoms between seizures.

Epilepsy is usually treated by medication and in some cases by surgery, devices or dietary changes.

EPILEPSY DIET RECIPES

BREAKFAS

1. Keto Sausage Gravy

Prep Time: 5 Minutes

Cook Time: 15 Minutes

Servings: 3

Ingredients

- 1 lb Ground Pork
- 2 Tablespoons Butter
- 2 tsp garlic powder
- 1 tsp onion powder
- 1/4 cup Almond Flour
- 2 cups Heavy Cream, may add more if you prefer a thinner gravy
- Salt and Pepper, to taste

Instructions

1. Cook ground pork in a skillet over medium-high heat for 10-15 minutes, until cooked through and at desired doneness.
2. Stir in the butter, garlic powder, and onion powder. Cook for two minutes more, stirring occasionally.
3. Sprinkle in the almond flour and stir until well combined.
4. Add the heavy cream and simmer over low heat for 8 minutes until thickened, adding additional cream as desired.
5. Season to taste with salt and pepper.

Prep Time: 15 Minutes

Cook Time: 10 Minutes

Servings: 6

Ingredients

- 1 lb salmon, cut into large chunks
- 6 oz pineapple, about ⅓ of a fresh pineapple, chopped into large chunks
- 1 red onion, medium, cut into large pieces
- 1 bell pepper, medium, any color, cut into large pieces
- 1 zucchini, medium, cut into large chunks
- Fresh cilantro, for garnish
- lime wedges, for garnish
- For Teriyaki Sauce
- ½ cup soy sauce, or coconut aminos
- 2 tbsp ginger paste
- 2 tbsp rice vinegar
- 2 tbsp stevia brown sugar
- 3 cloves garlic minced
- 2 tsp sesame oil
- 2 tsp Sriracha sauce

- salt and pepper, to taste

Instructions

1. In a small bowl, combine ingredients for the teriyaki marinade. Whisk to combine, and set aside. Heat the grill.
2. Assemble the skewers. On each wooden skewer, thread several pieces of salmon, pineapple, bell pepper, zucchini and onion. You can use more or less skewers as needed.
3. Brush the teriyaki marinade onto the salmon kebabs, coating all of the salmon and veggies. Reserve remaining marinade.
4. Place the salmon kebabs on the hot grill. Grill for 3-4 minutes on each side, turning once, or until salmon is just cooked through and veggies are slightly tender. Brush occasionally with extra marinade.
5. Remove skewers from the grill (carefully!). Brush with extra marinade, if desired. Serve with the lime wedges and cilantro.

Prep Time: 10 Minutes

Cook Time: 30 Minutes

Servings: 4

Ingredients

For the keto bang bang sauce:

- 1/2 cup mayo
- 1 tbsp sriracha, add additional tbsp for extra spicy
- 2 tsp chili garlic sauce
- 1 tsp rice vinegar
- 1 tbsp keto honey, or allulose sweetener
- salt and pepper, to taste

For the shrimp:

- 1 lb shrimp, peeled and deveined
- 1 egg
- 1/2 cup almond flour
- 2 tbsp parmesan cheese, grated
- salt and pepper, to taste
- Oil for frying
- Green onion and/or salad greens, optional for serving

Instructions

1. In a small bowl, stir together all of the ingredients for the keto bang bang sauce, until well combined. Set aside.
2. In one mixing bowl, crack the egg and lightly beat with a fork. Set aside.
3. In another mixing bowl, combine the almond four, parmesan, salt and pepper.
4. Heat 1-2 inches of oil in a heavy bottom pan over medium heat.
5. Dunk each piece of shrimp in the beaten egg, then dredge in the almond flour mixture.
6. Fry the shrimp in the oil for 3-4 minutes each side, or until cooked through. Repeat, working in batches, until all shrimps are fried.
7. Drain the shrimp on a layer of paper towels, then transfer to a clean mixing bowl.
8. Toss the shrimp with the bang bang sauce until lightly coated.
9. Garnish with the green onions and serve over salad greens, if desired.

Prep Time: 10 Minutes

Cook Time: 5 Minutes

Servings: 11

Ingredients

- 4 oz. of Melted Cream Cheese
- 1 and ½ cups of Whole Milk
- 2 Eggs
- 1 and ¾ cups of Almond Flour
- 3 teaspoons of Baking Powder
- couple dashes of Salt
- 3 teaspoons of Oil, such as sunflower oil
- 1 cup of Diced Strawberries
- Cooking Spray
- Diced Strawberries (for topping)

Instructions

1. Start by adding all your ingredients except your diced strawberries to your mixing bowl.
2. Mix on high until smooth.

3. Add one cup of strawberries, and fold into batter.

4. Grease your waffle maker.

5. Pour batter into your waffle maker.

6. Cook for 3 to 5 minutes.

7. Top with chopped strawberries.

8. Serve with syrup or whip cream and enjoy!

Prep Time: 20 Minutes

Cook Time: 60 Minutes

Servings: 10

Ingredients

- 2 pounds fully cooked rotisserie chicken
- 2 celery stalks, chopped
- 1 red bell pepper, diced
- 1/2 red onion, small, diced
- 1 teaspoon garlic powder
- 1 teaspoon paprika
- 1/4 teaspoon kosher salt
- 1 teaspoon black pepper
- 1 teaspoon dijon mustard
- 1 tablespoon lemon juice
- 2 teaspoons dill, fresh, chopped
- 1 tablespoon parsley, fresh, chopped
- 1/4 cup scallions, sliced
- 1/2 cup mayonnaise
- 1/2 avocado, peeled and pit removed

Instructions

1. Add the celery, bell pepper, and onion to a mixing bowl. Add the garlic, paprika, salt, pepper, mustard, lemon juice, dill, parsley, and mayonnaise to the bowl and stir to combine.

2. In a separate small bowl, mash the avocado with a fork until it is smooth and creamy.

3. Add the avocado to the vegetable mixture and fold together until combined.

4. Use a fork to shred the meat from the rotisserie chicken. Place the meat on a cutting board (leaving the skin behind) and roughly chop with a sharp knife.

5. Add the chopped chicken into the mixing bowl with the veggie mixture and stir until well combined.

6. Chill the chicken salad for 1 hour before serving. Top with scallions for garnish, if desired.

Prep Time: 30 Minutes

Cook Time: 30 Minutes

Servings: 4

Ingredients

For the crab cakes:

- 8 oz Lump Crab Meat
- 1 cup pork rind crumbs, or keto bread crumbs
- 1 egg
- ¼ cup scallions, chopped
- 1 tsp Dijon mustard
- 2 Tbsp Mayonnaise
- 1 tsp Old Bay seasoning
- Salt and pepper, to taste
- Oil, for frying

For topping the crab cakes:

- 16 Asparagus spears
- 4 eggs poached
- Salt and pepper, to taste

For the hollandaise sauce:

- 4 Egg yolks, beaten
- 2 Tbsp Heavy whipping cream
- 8 Tbsp Butter, unsalted
- 2 tbsp fresh lemon juice
- Salt, to taste

Instructions

1. Place one egg into a small bowl and beat lightly.
2. In a large mixing bowl, combine the crab meat, pork rind crumbs (or keto breadcrumbs), beaten egg, scallions, Dijon mustard, mayonnaise, old bay seasoning, salt, and pepper. Mix until well combined. Knead with your hands to fully combine, if needed.
3. Form the crab cake mixture into four evenly sized patties.
4. Heat a thin layer of oil in a skillet over medium high heat. Add the crab cakes and fry for 3-4 minutes on each side, until crispy and lightly golden.
5. Remove the crab cakes from the pan, and set them aside on a paper towel lined plate to drain.
6. Pour most of the oil out of the skillet, reduce the heat to medium, and saute the asparagus for 6-7 minutes

until crisp tender. Add salt and pepper, to taste. Set aside.

7. To poach the eggs: Bring a medium sized pot of water to a boil. Reduce to a simmer. Carefully crack the eggs into the hot water, taking care not to break the yolk. Cook for 2-3 minutes until the egg white is set and the eggs are cooked to your liking, and remove from the water with a slotted spoon. Set aside.

8. To make the hollandaise sauce: Add the butter to a saucepan and heat over medium heat. When butter is just melted, add the whipping cream and lemon juice. Stir to combine. Remove from the heat and slowly add the egg yolks, whisking continuously until the sauce is smooth and thick. Add salt to taste. Be careful not to heat the egg yolks too much, or they will scramble!

9. To serve, top each crab cake with a few pieces of asparagus and a poached egg. Drizzle with the hollandaise sauce.

Prep Time: 10 Minutes

Cook Time: 10 Minutes

Servings: 12

Ingredients

1 8 oz. Block cream cheese, softened

½ cup Greek yogurt

1 cup shredded cheddar cheese

Dried apricots, cut into fine bits

5 slices cooked bacon, crumbled into fine bits (best if cooked crispy)

1/3 cup everything bagel seasoning

12-15 pretzel sticks

Instructions

1. In a medium-sized bowl, cream together cream cheese, Greek yogurt and cheddar cheese. Mix until all three ingredients are well-combined.

2. Fold in apricot bits and bacon. Mix thoroughly.

3. Pour everything bagel seasoning into a bowl.

4. Line a baking sheet or cutting board with wax paper. Roll the cheese mixture into small spheres, about 1 ½ inches in diameter.

5. Roll each cheeseball into the seasoning, coating it evenly.

6. Place gently on lined working surface. Insert one pretzel stick at the top center of each cheeseball.

7. Serve and enjoy! Pairs very well with crackers.

Prep Time: 10 Minutes

Cook Time: 30 Minutes

Servings: 4

Ingredients

Nonstick cooking spray:

- 1 lb skinless chicken breasts, cubed
- 10 oz fresh baby spinach
- 8 oz cream cheese, softened
- ¾ cup shredded mozzarella cheese, divided
- ¼ cup sour cream
- 2 tsp minced garlic or garlic paste
- Salt and black pepper

Instructions

1. Preheat the oven to 400°F. Coat a 9x13" baking dish with cooking spray.
2. Spread out the chicken in the dish. Layer the spinach over the top, keeping it as flat as possible.

3. In a medium bowl, combine the cream cheese, ¼ cup of mozzarella, the sour cream, and garlic. Season

4. With salt and pepper to taste. Spoon the mixture on top of the spinach.

5. Cover with kitchen foil and bake for 20 minutes. Remove from the oven, uncover, and top with the

6. Remaining ½ cup of mozzarella.

7. Bake for another 10 to 15 minutes, until the chicken has reached an internal temperature of 165°F.

9. Easy Low Carb Pecan Cookies

Prep Time: 5 Minutes

Cook Time: 10 Minutes

Servings: 12

Ingredients

- 1 cup chopped pecans
- 1 egg
- ¼ cup Lakanto, or similar sweetener

Instructions

1. Preheat the oven to 350F.
2. Grind the pecans as finely as possible using a food processor.
3. Break the egg into a bowl and whisk until lightly beaten. Add the pecans and sweetener, then mix well.
4. Divide the mixture into 12, then place each portion onto a baking tray lined with a silicone mat.
5. Bake for 8-10 minutes until firm. Leave to cool slightly then transfer to a cooling rack.
6. When completely cool, store in an airtight container.

Prep Time: 5 Minutes

Cook Time: 5 Minutes

Servings: 1

Ingredients

- fl oz unsweetened tomato juice
- 2 tbs vodka
- 1 tsp Worcestershire sauce
- 1 tsp lemon juice
- 2-3 drops hot sauce, or to taste
- Salt and pepper
- Ice
- Various garnishes, as desired

Instructions

1. Mix together the tomato juice, vodka, Worcestershire sauce, lemon juice, hot sauce, salt and pepper.
2. Pour the cocktail over a glass filled with ice, and garnish as desired.

3. Note: If you want to make a seasoned rim for the glass, mix a little paprika in with some salt on a small plate. Run a wedge of lemon around the edge of the glass, then dip it in the salt mixture.

11. Keto Fried Queso Fresco

Prep Time: 5 Minutes

Cook Time: 8 Minutes

Servings: 4

Ingredients

- 10 oz round of queso fresco
- 1 tbs olive oil
- ¼ cup low carb salsa

Instructions

1. Cut a round of queso fresco into slices. Cut the very longest ones in half to make them easier to handle.
2. Heat some olive oil in a large skillet over a medium-high heat. Add the slices of cheese to the hot pan (I had to cook mine in two batches). After a minute or two, flip them all over.
3. Then after another couple of minutes, remove them from the skillet and drain on some paper towels.

4. As they cool they will firm up a little, which makes them easier to handle. But make sure they are still warm when you serve them.

Prep Time: 5 Minutes

Cook Time: 2 Minutes

Servings: 4

Ingredients

- 1½ cups (150g) shredded mozzarella
- 2 tbs (31g) cream cheese
- 1 cup (115g / 4 oz) fine almond flour
- 1 egg, beaten

Instructions

1. Place the mozzarella and cream cheese in a medium size microwaveable bowl.
2. Microwave for 1 minute, stir and then cook for another 30 seconds.
3. Stir in the almond flour and beaten egg.
4. Let the dough cool slightly, then knead until smooth. Add a little extra almond flour if the dough is too sticky, then knead again.

Prep Time: 5 Minutes

Cook Time: 6 Minutes

Servings: 4

Ingredients

- 1 tbs butter
- 1 tsp olive oil
- 1 lb calamari (squid) tubes and tentacles, fully defrosted if previously frozen
- 1 tsp garlic paste or minced garlic
- 1 tsp lemon juice
- salt and pepper
- 1 tbs chopped parsley

Instructions

1. Heat the butter and oil together in a large skillet.
2. Cut the squid tubes into rings and add them to the skillet, together with the tentacles and the garlic.
3. Continue to cook until the calamari has firmed up, about 5 minutes.

4. Add the lemon juice, salt and pepper. Use a slotted spoon to transfer the calamari to a serving dish.

5. Garnish with the parsley, more black pepper, and an extra squeeze of lemon.

Prep Time: 5 Minutes

Cook Time: 20 Minutes

Servings: 2

Ingredients

- 1 tbs olive oil
- 1 tsp onion powder
- 1 lb ground turkey
- 1 red bell pepper, deseeded and diced
- 1 tsp dried oregano
- 1 tsp paprika
- 1 tsp ground cumin
- ½ cup shredded Mexican blend cheese
- Fresh cilantro, chopped
- Sour cream, shredded lettuce and/or low carb wraps for serving

Instructions

1. Heat the oil in a large skillet. Add ground turkey and onion powder. Sauté until the meat has browned.

2. Add paprika, ground cumin, dried oregano and chopped red bell pepper. Continue to cook until the pepper has softened.

3. Sprinkle over the shredded cheese and cook until the cheese has melted. Remove from the heat and scatter over some chopped fresh cilantro.

4. Serve with shredded lettuce, sour cream, and/or low carb wraps!

Prep Time: 20 Minutes

Cook Time: 20 Minutes

Servings: 4

Ingredients

- 6 stalks fresh rhubarb, roughly chopped
- 1 tsp Lakanto, or similar sweetener
- 2 tbs water
- ½ cup almond flour
- ¼ cup flaxseed meal
- 3 tbs Lakanto
- 2 tbs unsalted butter

Instructions

1. Preheat the oven to 375F.
2. Add the rhubarb, sweetener and water to a saucepan and simmer until rhubarb is cooked.
3. Meanwhile, make the crumble topping by rubbing together the remaining ingredients until they are the size of large breadcrumbs.

4. Test the rhubarb for sweetness and adjust if necessary, then spread it over the base of a small baking dish.

5. Sprinkle the topping over the rhubarb and bake for 15-20 minutes or until golden brown on top and the rhubarb is bubbling through the topping.

Prep Time: 5 Minutes

Cook Time: 12 Minutes

Servings: 8

Ingredients

- 2 eggs
- ½ cup shredded cheddar cheese
- ¼ cup shredded mozzarella
- ¼ cup shredded Parmesan
- ½ cup almond flour
- ½ tsp baking powder
- black pepper

Instructions

1. Preheat the oven to 400F.
2. Add the eggs to a large bowl and whisk until lightly beaten.
3. Add the remaining ingredients and mix well.

4. Divide the mixture into 8 sections, roll each section into a ball and place it on a baking sheet lined with baking parchment or a silicone mat.

5. Bake for 10-12 minutes until golden brown.

Prep Time: 5 Minutes

Cook Time: 30 Minutes

Servings: 4

Ingredients

- 2 large turnips
- 6 tbs oil, divided
- 2 tsp onion powder
- ½ tsp paprika
- salt and pepper
- fresh thyme or parsley, optional

Instructions

1. Preheat the oven to 425F.
2. Peel the turnips and cut it into matchsticks.
3. Add 2 tbs of the oil, onion powder and paprika to a bag or bowl, then add the turnip. Turn to coat in the mixture.
4. Add the remaining oil to a baking pan and place in the oven for 5 minutes.

5. Carefully add the turnip to the hot oil, then season with salt and pepper.

6. Roast for 25 minutes or until starting to get crispy.

7. To garnish, sprinkle some fresh herbs like thyme or parsley over the top.

Prep Time: 5 Minutes

Cook Time: 5 Minutes

Servings: 4

Ingredients

- 0.3 oz packet of sugar free jello, any flavor
- 1 envelope unflavored powdered gelatin, 1 envelope = 0.25 oz/7.4g
- ¼ - ⅓ cup cold water

Instructions

1. Add all three ingredients to a small saucepan, stir well, and cook over a low heat.
2. Cook until all the granules have dissolved - approx 2-3 minutes.
3. Use a jug, squeeze bottle or a spoon to carefully pour the mixture into a silicone mold.
4. Place the filled mold on something firm like a small chopping board (to stop the mold twisting). Let the

jello cool then place in the fridge for 30-40 minutes until set.

Prep Time: 8 Minutes

Cook Time: 8 Minutes

Servings: 4

Ingredients

- ½ cup (4 oz) cream cheese
- ½ cup heavy cream
- ¼ cup water
- 1 egg yolk
- salt and pepper, to taste

Instructions

1. Add the cream cheese, cream and water to a saucepan and cook over a low heat until the cream cheese has melted.
2. Temper the egg yolk by adding a little of the cream sauce to it, mixing well, then adding the yolk back into the cream mixture.
3. Stir constantly over a low heat for a few minutes until the sauce has thickened.

4. Season with salt and pepper to taste.

Prep Time: 5 Minutes

Cook Time: 25 Minutes

Servings: 6

Ingredients

- 4-6 chicken thighs
- 1/4 cup hot sauce, such as Frank's Red Hot
- 1/2 cup mayonnaise
- 1/4 cup Parmesan cheese, grated
- 1 teaspoon garlic powder
- 1/3 cup Keto breadcrumbs, homemade or store bought

Instructions

1. Preheat the oven to 425F degrees.
2. Arrange the chicken thighs in an 8" x 8" baking dish.
3. Pour the hot sauce over the chicken thighs, and set aside.
4. In a small bowl, mix together the mayonnaise, Parmesan and garlic powder.

5. Spread the mayonnaise mixture evenly over the top of the chicken. Sprinkle with the keto-friendly breadcrumbs.

6. Bake 20-25 minutes, until the top is golden brown, or until an inserted meat thermometer reads 165F.

21. Keto Cilantro Chicken

Prep Time: 10 Minutes

Cook Time: 20 Minutes

Servings: 3

Ingredients

- ¼ cup fresh cilantro leaves
- 2 tbs lime juice
- 2 tbs soy sauce (or tamari)
- 1 tbs ginger paste
- 1 tsp garlic paste
- 1 serrano or jalapeño pepper, deseeded and roughly diced, optional
- ½ cup unsweetened canned coconut milk
- 1 lb skinless, boneless chicken thighs (about 6)
- salt and black pepper
- cilantro sprigs, to garnish

Instructions

1. Prepare the marinade by adding the cilantro, garlic, ginger, lime juice, soy sauce, and pepper (if using) to a small food processor, and blend until smooth.
2. Stir in the coconut milk, and pour it over the chicken. Cover and marinate in the fridge for at least an hour.
3. Preheat a grill or grill pan over a medium-high heat, and cook the chicken until cooked through, turning as needed. Season with salt and black pepper.
4. Meanwhile, bring the marinade to a boil and allow it to reduce. Do NOT skip this step if you want to serve the marinade as a sauce.
5. Transfer the cooked chicken to a serving plate, and pour the reduced marinade over. Garnish with cilantro sprigs.

Prep Time: 5 Minutes

Cook Time: 30 Minutes

Servings: 2

Ingredients

- non-stick spray
- 2 chicken breasts, cut into bite-sized pieces
- ¼ cup dry white wine (or chicken broth)
- 1 tbs garlic paste
- 1 tbs Dijon mustard
- 1 tbs dried oregano
- 14 oz can baby artichoke hearts, drained
- salt and black pepper
- 1 lemon, sliced

Instructions

1. Preheat the oven to 375 F (190C).
2. Spray a large baking dish with non-stick spray, and add the chicken.

3. In a bowl, mix together some dry white wine (or chicken broth), garlic paste, Dijon mustard, and dried oregano.

4. Pour the mixture over the chicken, then add some baby artichoke hearts. Season everything well with salt and black pepper.

5. Place some slices of lemon over the top, then roast for 30 minutes or until the chicken reaches an internal temperature of 165F.

6. Use a slotted spoon to serve the chicken and artichokes, then drizzle a little of the cooking liquid over the top.

Prep Time: 5 Minutes

Cook Time: 10 Minutes

Servings: 2

Ingredients

- 2 tbs unsalted butter
- juice of half a lemon
- 2 x 6 oz cod fillets (chopped into bite-sized pieces, optional)
- salt and black pepper
- ¼ cup fresh basil leaves, sliced
- lemon slices, to garnish

Instructions

1. Melt the butter in a small cast iron pan over a medium heat. Whisk in the lemon juice.
2. Add the cod, season with salt and black pepper, and turn to coat in the lemon butter.
3. When the fish is cooked through, stir in some sliced basil leaves and allow them to wilt,

4. Serve, garnished with the lemon slices.

Prep Time: 15 Minutes

Cook Time: 40 Minutes

Servings: 4

Ingredients

- 4 large jalapeños (approx 5" long)
- 4 oz cream cheese, softened
- 1 cup shredded sharp cheddar cheese
- black pepper
- 1 lb ground sausage or pork
- 4 slices bacon

Instructions

1. Preheat the oven to 375 F (190C)
2. Prepare the jalapeños by cutting a slit along the pepper lengthwise, then using an upturned teaspoon to scoop out the membranes and seeds.
3. In a bowl, mix together the softened cream cheese, shredded sharp cheddar cheese, and black pepper.

4. Scoop the cheese mixture into the jalapeños - this can get a little messy!

5. Divide the ground sausage or pork into four sections, then wrap the jalapeños completely in the meat. Try and keep the slit of the jalapeños facing up.

6. Finally, wrap each "egg" in a strip of bacon, secure it with a couple of toothpicks, and place them on a baking sheet lined with a baking rack.

7. Roast for 35-40 minutes or until the pork is full cooked and the bacon is crispy.

8. Remove the toothpicks before serving.

Prep Time: 5 Minutes

Cook Time: 15 Minutes

Servings: 3

Ingredients

- 1 lb Ground Pork
- 2 Tablespoons Butter
- 2 tsp garlic powder
- 1 tsp onion powder
- 1/4 cup Almond Flour
- 2 cups Heavy Cream, may add more if you prefer a thinner gravy
- Salt and Pepper, to taste

Instructions

1. Cook ground pork in a skillet over medium-high heat for 10-15 minutes, until cooked through and at desired doneness.
2. Stir in the butter, garlic powder, and onion powder. Cook for two minutes more, stirring occasionally.

3. Sprinkle in the almond flour and stir until well combined.

4. Add the heavy cream and simmer over low heat for 8 minutes until thickened, adding additional cream as desired.

5. Season to taste with salt and pepper.

Prep Time: 10 Minutes

Cook Time: 30 Minutes

Servings: 4

Ingredients

For the keto bang bang sauce:

- 1/2 cup mayo
- 1 tbsp sriracha, add additional tbsp for extra spicy
- 2 tsp chili garlic sauce
- 1 tsp rice vinegar
- 1 tbsp keto honey, or allulose sweetener
- salt and pepper, to taste

For the shrimp:

- 1 lb shrimp, peeled and deveined
- 1 egg
- 1/2 cup almond flour
- 2 tbsp parmesan cheese, grated
- salt and pepper, to taste
- Oil for frying
- Green onion and/or salad greens, optional for serving

Instructions

1. In a small bowl, stir together all of the ingredients for the keto bang bang sauce, until well combined. Set aside.
2. In one mixing bowl, crack the egg and lightly beat with a fork. Set aside.
3. In another mixing bowl, combine the almond four, parmesan, salt and pepper.
4. Heat 1-2 inches of oil in a heavy bottom pan over medium heat.
5. Dunk each piece of shrimp in the beaten egg, then dredge in the almond flour mixture.
6. Fry the shrimp in the oil for 3-4 minutes each side, or until cooked through. Repeat, working in batches, until all shrimps are fried.
7. Drain the shrimp on a layer of paper towels, then transfer to a clean mixing bowl.
8. Toss the shrimp with the bang bang sauce until lightly coated.
9. Garnish with the green onions and serve over salad greens, if desired.

Prep Time: 20 Minutes

Cook Time: 60 Minutes

Servings: 10

Ingredients

- 2 pounds fully cooked rotisserie chicken
- 2 celery stalks, chopped
- 1 red bell pepper, diced
- 1/2 red onion, small, diced
- 1 teaspoon garlic powder
- 1 teaspoon paprika
- 1/4 teaspoon kosher salt
- 1 teaspoon black pepper
- 1 teaspoon dijon mustard
- 1 tablespoon lemon juice
- 2 teaspoons dill, fresh, chopped
- 1 tablespoon parsley, fresh, chopped
- 1/4 cup scallions, sliced
- 1/2 cup mayonnaise
- 1/2 avocado, peeled and pit removed

Instructions

1. Add the celery, bell pepper, and onion to a mixing bowl. Add the garlic, paprika, salt, pepper, mustard, lemon juice, dill, parsley, and mayonnaise to the bowl and stir to combine.

2. In a separate small bowl, mash the avocado with a fork until it is smooth and creamy.

3. Add the avocado to the vegetable mixture and fold together until combined.

4. Use a fork to shred the meat from the rotisserie chicken. Place the meat on a cutting board (leaving the skin behind) and roughly chop with a sharp knife.

5. Add the chopped chicken into the mixing bowl with the veggie mixture and stir until well combined.

6. Chill the chicken salad for 1 hour before serving. Top with scallions for garnish, if desired.

Prep Time: 5 Minutes

Cook Time: 25 Minutes

Servings: 6

Ingredients

- 4-6 chicken thighs
- 1/4 cup hot sauce, such as Frank's Red Hot
- 1/2 cup mayonnaise
- 1/4 cup Parmesan cheese, grated
- 1 teaspoon garlic powder
- 1/3 cup Keto breadcrumbs, homemade or store bought

Instructions

1. Preheat the oven to 425F degrees.
2. Arrange the chicken thighs in an 8" x 8" baking dish.
3. Pour the hot sauce over the chicken thighs, and set aside.
4. In a small bowl, mix together the mayonnaise, Parmesan and garlic powder.

5. Spread the mayonnaise mixture evenly over the top of the chicken. Sprinkle with the keto-friendly breadcrumbs.

6. Bake 20-25 minutes, until the top is golden brown, or until an inserted meat thermometer reads 165F.

Prep Time: 15 Minutes

Cook Time: 45 Minutes

Servings: 4

Ingredients

- 1-2 tbs olive oil
- 2 pre-cooked Andouille sausage links, sliced
- 4 small skinless, boneless chicken thighs, cut into bite-sized pieces
- 1 tsp Cajun seasoning
- 1 rib of celery, chopped
- ½ orange or red bell pepper, seeded and chopped
- 1 tbs garlic paste or minced garlic
- ½ cup fresh or frozen chopped okra
- 1 cup chicken broth
- 10 oz cauliflower rice
- 1 tbs onion powder
- salt and black pepper, to taste
- 8 oz raw shrimp, peeled and deveined
- 2 green onions, finely chopped, to garnish

Instructions

1. Heat one tablespoon of the oil in a large high-sided skillet. Add the andouille sausage and cook for 5 minutes over a medium heat, turning frequently.

2. Use a slotted spoon to remove the sausage and set aside. Next, add the diced chicken, and turn to coat it in the oil. Sprinkle the Cajun seasoning over the chicken, then cook for ten minutes, turning occasionally.

3. Again, use the slotted spoon to remove the chicken. Splash some more oil in if needed, then add the celery and bell pepper. After five minutes, add the garlic and okra.

4. Return the sausage and chicken to the skillet, together with the chicken broth, cauliflower rice, and onion powder. Bring to the boil and then reduce to a fast simmer for 15-20 minutes or until the cauliflower is cooked and most of the liquid has been reduced.

5. Taste for seasoning and add more Cajun seasoning, and/or salt and black pepper as desired. Finally, add the raw shrimp and continue to cook until it is cooked through.

6. Garnish with d green onions.

Prep Time: 5 Minutes

Cook Time: 10 Minutes

Servings: 4

Ingredients

- 2 tbs olive oil
- 2 tsp garlic paste
- 1 bunch fresh asparagus (approx. 9 oz when trimmed)
- salt and black pepper
- 4 slices bacon, roughly chopped

Instructions

1. Preheat the oven to 400F.
2. Make the garlic oil by whisking the garlic paste into the oil in a large bowl.
3. Trim the woody ends from the asparagus and place them in the bowl. Toss to coat in the oil.
4. Transfer the asparagus to a baking sheet and season with salt and pepper.

5. Roast for 8-15 minutes, depending on thickness of the stalks and personal preference.
6. Meanwhile, roughly chop some bacon and fry it until crispy.
7. Place the asparagus on a serving platter, drain the cooked bacon on paper towels, and sprinkle the bacon over the asparagus.